Reaching for the Top in the Land Down Under

Marc Maurer
Editor

Large Type Edition

A KERNEL BOOK
published by
NATIONAL FEDERATION OF THE BLIND

ISBN 1-885218-22-2

Printed in the United States of America

Table of Contents

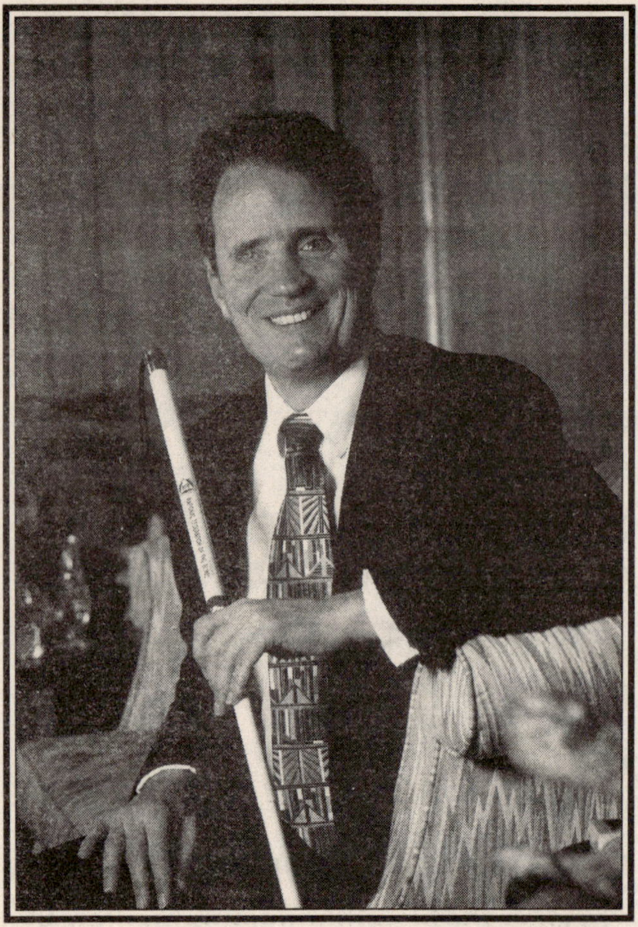

Marc Maurer, President
National Federation of the Blind

Editor's Introduction

This year we celebrate the tenth anniversary of the inauguration of the Kernel Book series. It is customary at the time of such milestones to look back and to look forward—to see where we have been and where we want to go.

Blindness is not the same for us as it was before we started sending the Kernel Books to people like you. This is so because blindness is no longer the same for you either, and this is what makes it different for us.

Let me explain. Through the Kernel Books you have come to know us. You know such things as that we need to be taught Braille when we are children in school, that we must learn to use a long white cane or a guide dog for mobility, and that there is special technology that is helpful to us.

You know that we want to be given the chance to try instead of always being told that we can't do whatever it is, and you know that belief—ours in ourselves and yours in us—is critical.

You have come to understand that very often the real problem of blindness is not the blindness itself but the mistaken notions and misunderstandings about blindness, which are so widely prevalent in society.

The very fact that tens of thousands of Kernel Book readers have come to have these new understandings about blindness is changing what blindness means for us as we live our daily lives. We find employers more likely to consider us for jobs and our neighbors more willing to include us in community activities. Where there was misunderstanding and frustration there is now welcome and friendship.

This volume, *Reaching for the Top in the Land Down Under,* is number twenty in the

Kernel Book series. It takes its name from the fact that I and a number of other blind leaders in the National Federation of the Blind traveled to Australia last fall to participate in the General Assembly of the World Blind Union.

That this journey took place at all perhaps illustrates the kind of change I am talking about, for there was a time in my life when I would have thought the very idea of my leading such an expedition was impossible. And certainly my sighted friends and associates would have thought so! This is the type of thing I mean when I say that blindness has changed for us, and that it has changed for you, too.

Revolution, the dictionary tells us, is "sudden or momentous change." By these standards I think it is fair to say that what we have achieved during these past ten years in writing, publishing, and distributing the Kernel Books is truly a revolution. For the change in the way blind people are regarded in the hearts and minds of our readers has been momentous, and equally so, the way we regard ourselves.

But, fear not. There is still a long enough way to go (for us who are blind and you who have come to share the journey with us) that I am sure there will be another decade of Kernel Books—for us to share. Together we will finish the journey.

Marc Maurer
Baltimore, Maryland
2001

WHY LARGE TYPE?

The type size used in this book is 14 point for two important reasons: One, because typesetting of 14 point or larger complies with federal standards for the printing of materials for visually impaired readers, and we want to show you what type size is helpful for people with limited sight.

The second reason is that many of our friends and supporters have asked us to print our paperback books in 14-point type so they too can easily read them. Many people with limited sight do not use Braille. We hope that by printing this book in a larger type than customary, many more people will be able to benefit from it.

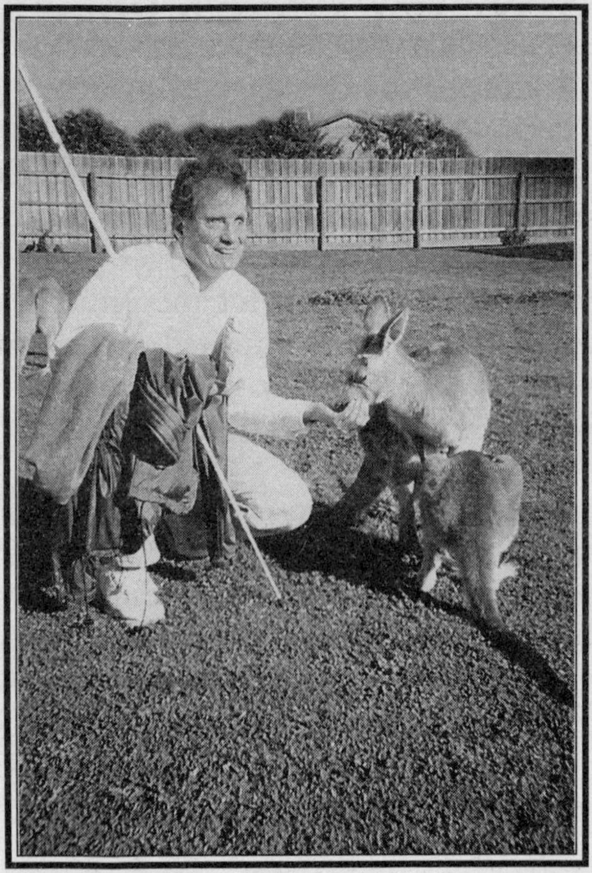

Marc Maurer

Reaching for the Top in the Land Down Under

by Marc Maurer

In a film entitled *The Music Man*, produced in the 1960's, there is a song which asks, "How can there be any sin in sincere?" The question is, of course, a play on words; *sin* and *sincere* sound alike, but they are unrelated. However, the question has even greater significance.

Sincere is derived from the two Latin words "sine" and "cere"—meaning without wax. It appears that sneakiness and fraud have been with us a long time. The ancient myth tells us that Roman sculptors were not as good at using the strength of stone as their Greek counterparts. Greek statuary was often graceful, but the Romans (who were trying to imitate this art form) carved figures in stone that were not strong enough to support their own weight. Consequently, many of the Roman sculptures cracked. Some sculptors filled these cracks with wax to make their statues appear to be complete and perfect.

Because this practice came to be widespread, the legend "sine cere" (without wax) became a mark of excellence because the statues had no cracks. Hence, we have the word sincere, which has come to mean genuine—without pretension or hidden flaw.

Within the National Federation of the Blind we try to meet the standard of sincerity; we try to build opportunity for the blind which will meet realistic tests of value and worth; and we are making progress. In fact, many of us have gained such encouragement from our blind brothers and sisters and from our sighted friends that we concentrate more on the ordinary demands of living than we do on blindness itself.

The National Federation of the Blind participates in a world organization called the World Blind Union, which is a collection of groups from more than 150 countries engaged in activities to promote opportunity for the blind. I am one of the delegates. Once every four years a gathering of these delegates occurs; the most recent meeting took place in Melbourne, Australia, in the fall of 2000.

I participate in these meetings to let people know what we are doing in the United States, to encourage Braille literacy for blind children, and to help blind adults get jobs. I encourage people in other lands to learn what they can from us, and I try to learn from them. I also put my mind to forming international friendships with people who recognize that the talent of the blind should be used so that we can work with each other across international borders.

Melbourne, Australia, is halfway around the world from my home in Baltimore,

Maryland. The international gathering planned around the General Assembly of the World Blind Union would take place over a period of more than a week.

Because I would be gone from my family for such a lengthy period, and because studying a foreign culture and continent would be interesting, I decided to invite my two children, David and Dianna, to accompany me and my wife Patricia to Australia.

As Kernel Book readers know, my wife Patricia and I are both blind, and our children are sighted. In planning the trip to Australia, I considered activities that all of us would enjoy. When I visit a new country, I like to examine the customs and daily activities of the inhabitants. I try the food, and I visit the monuments that are recommended to the tourists. However, I also like to learn about the local shops and the daily routine for people in that part of the world.

When I informed David and Dianna that they were traveling with us to Australia, they were delighted and dubious at the same time. A trip to an unknown place is a great pleasure, but they were fearful of the consequences of their being out of school for two whole weeks.

David is a junior in high school. He has sometimes excelled academically, but sometimes his performance has been mediocre. There were even times when his teachers warned us that he had better put more effort into his work, or he would fail.

We had a family discussion about the upcoming trip, and we talked about the need for David and Dianna to do their schoolwork while we traveled. They urged me to consider leaving them home so that they wouldn't get behind in their studies. However, we eventually came to the conclusion that the four Maurers would go and that the two younger Maurers would spend part of each day hitting the books.

I made David a proposal, which I thought might intrigue him. He loves automobiles. I suspect he thinks that they help to define the personality of the people who drive them. I said to him that if he achieved straight A's in his schoolwork for two consecutive academic quarters, I would let him pick out the car of his choice that we would buy and that he could drive.

Until the spring of 2000, the Maurers had never owned an automobile. David and his mom persuaded me to buy one, which found its way into our driveway on David's sixteenth birthday. David was first astonished, then pleased, then disappointed with the car—a 1994 Chrysler New Yorker. He thought it was an "old man's car." He wanted something sportier, he said.

Sometimes he wanted a Volkswagen GTI; sometimes it was a Honda Civic (or maybe a Prelude), and sometimes it was a Lexus. Often he wanted something else—sometimes a 1964 Impala. However, as he drove the Chrysler he came to like it. It was peppier than many of the cars driven by his friends, and the Chrysler is big enough to carry six passengers—or even more if you are willing to squeeze.

Even so, David wanted a different car; I told him he could have one if he got the grades. The only condition placed on the deal was that I had to be able to afford it.

After this proposal had been made to him, David's behavior changed. He began planning for the new car. He considered what color he wanted, what kind of engine would be needed, and what type of stereo system he would buy for it. He was quite certain that he would need a stick shift and that he would want to modify the suspension.

I told him that buying the car would be my responsibility and that all other expenses of modifying it would be in his domain. He asked me if he was required to get A's on all of his tests. I responded that this was not essential but that an A average for his overall grade in every subject would be required.

It is one long haul from Baltimore to Melbourne. The first leg of the trip takes you from Baltimore to Los Angeles. Then, there are 15 hours in the air from Los Angeles to Australia. It seemed that every seat on our plane was full, and after awhile I found it difficult to find any way to relax. Every hour or two I climbed out of the seat ostensibly to search out a bathroom. However, the real reason was to find someplace to stretch; airplane seats are not built for long hours.

Travel to Australia from the West Coast of the United States involves crossing the International Dateline. We left on Thursday evening, flying for 15 hours, and we arrived on Saturday morning. We lost all of Friday. Tired from the long trip, we headed from the airport to the hotel. David Maurer was fascinated by the traffic patterns.

People in Australia drive on the left; the steering wheels in cars are placed on the right. Traffic patterns for changing lanes and turning right are complex, and David felt that he should offer advice.

During all of the time that we spent in this interesting, friendly country, David looked at the cars comparing them to the ones in the United States and deciding which would be the most desirable for him to own. Most of them were smaller than the ones in our own country; the Australians referred to the large American built machine affectionately as the "yank tank."

The climate in Australia is moderate to hot. Melbourne is on the southern coast, in the more temperate part of the country, and November is the beginning of the Australian spring. Australia has two territories and six states. The island of Tasmania, situated south of the main continent, is one of them. The country itself is approxmiately the same size as the United

States, but it has only about 19 million inhabitants—less than ten percent of the population of our country. Ninety-six percent of the land cannot produce crops because it is too dry.

The population is clustered along the coast in an area shaped rather like a boomerang. The interior of Australia may become very, very hot during the "summer months" in January and February, reaching temperatures of more than 125 degrees.

The parts of the country which have not been substantially settled are known as the "outback." In many parts of the outback, the land stretches for miles with nobody on it, with no town, and with no roads. Fortunately, we were along the southern coast in a lush, green, populated area.

As I have said, when I visit another country, I taste the food. In Australia they serve the "Aussie Burger," which at McDonald's is called the "McOz." It consists of a hamburger served on a bun along with lettuce, tomatoes, cheese, beets, a fried egg, and a slice of pineapple.

I think (but I am not certain) that the slice of pineapple is a recent innovation. However, I believe that the meat, beets, and fried egg are of long standing. I ate an excellent version at a fish and chips place. I also tried the McOz, but there was too much sauce for my taste, and red beet juice kept dripping off my bun.

On the streets of Melbourne there are small cafes with sidewalk tables. Each morning before the meetings began, we stopped for breakfast. Some of the items on the menu were beans on toast, spaghetti on toast, and shark. On separate mornings I tried the beans and the shark— both good. I also tried a thing called a lamb fry, which was liver on toast. I was pleased to have had it, but I thought once was enough.

The coffee was universally good. Each cup was brewed individually with a strong, robust, aromatic flavor without bitterness or unseemly assertiveness. People of the United States do many things well, but the Australians seem to have captured the spirit of coffee. No matter where we ordered the brew—from the most elegant restaurant to the lowliest lunch counter, it tasted delectable.

Australia has a flourishing wine business. We visited the Seppelt Winery, which has thousands upon thousands of bottles of wine stored in underground caverns excavated by out-of-work miners, who were left without employment after the Australian gold rush came to an end in the later part of the 19th century.

The ceilings and walls of many of the caverns are covered with a thick layer of black mold, which adds both to the atmosphere and to the aroma of the cool, dank cellars. Although the wine industry of Australia is not as old as that of France and probably not as old as that of California, it produces some excellent robust wines, of which Australia is justifiably proud.

Australia is known for kangaroos. We visited a wildlife preserve where there was a wombat, some koala bears, and many small kangaroos—which some people said were wallabies. Baby kangaroos, known as joeys, ride in their mother's pouches, where they can nurse.

The operator of the wildlife prescrve informed us that a female kangaroo can have a half-grown young one, a joey, and a yet-to-be-born infant all at the same time. If food and water become sparse, the yet to be born kangaroo will stop developing until its mother finds enough sustenance to permit it to continue to grow. The kangaroos I met were quite friendly, and I fed them from the palm of my hand.

A large colony of diminutive penguins lives on Phillip Island 50 or 60 miles from Melbourne. As many as 10,000 come home at dusk crossing the beach in a "penguin parade" from fishing expeditions in the sea. The penguins are about 18 inches long, and they sometimes eat so much fish that they fall over when returning to their burrows.

Two penguins live in each burrow, and one swims out to sea to fish while the other stays at home. A penguin may be at sea hunting fish for two or three days at a time, but when it comes home, it shares its fish with its mate.

The ranger on duty at Phillip Island had a penguin in a box. He asked me if I wanted to touch it, and I put my hand through a hole in the box. The penguin moved, and I was startled until I realized that the ranger was wiggling the box to make me believe the penguin was still alive. The penguin had been stuffed so members of the public could study it at close range. It is not practical to touch them in their native habitat.

David and Dianna were charmed by the creatures; David wanted to take one home. However, the ranger told us that there is a $20,000 fine for disturbing the penguins and that they smell strongly of fish anyway, so David would not want one.

He also told us that there is a severe fine for taking pictures of the birds. They cross the beach about an hour after sunset, and the flash from a camera blinds them for three or four days. The blinded penguins get lost and wander aimlessly without being able to locate their burrows. Only the most specialized cameras that can take pictures in twilight without additional light can be used to film the penguin parade.

We were invited to the home of an Australian family for dinner. It was a jolly gathering with much the same spirit that a dinner party might have in the United States. We had salad, lasagna, and chocolate cake.

Sometimes when people come to the Maurer household in our country, we entertain them with a barbecued supper. Occasionally we cook hot dogs. Under those circumstances we might sing the Armour hot dog song, which most of our guests don't seem to remember. We had been visiting the tourist sights in Melbourne. One of them is a building where Vegemite was manufactured.

Vegemite is a yeast product that was invented in the 1920's during a time when wholesome food was in short supply. We mentioned observing the Vegemite production plant, and our hosts offered us a taste of this concoction along with a rendition of the Vegemite song.

Vegemite may have approximately the same position in Australia that peanut butter has in the United States. It is a yeasty, salty substance to be spread on a slice of bread. We were coaxed through the process. First the bread is to be spread with a small amount of butter or margarine. Then Vegemite is applied very sparingly. My host told me to take an amount on the tip of my knife approximately the size of a button— this would be quite sufficient. When spread thinly over the butter, the Vegemite produced a powerful but tasty flavor.

For those who have not heard the Armour hot dog song or the Vegemite song, here they are:

The Armour Hot Dog Song

Hot dogs, Armour hot dogs
What kinds of kids love Armour hot dogs?
Big kids, little kids, kids who climb on rocks
Fat kids, skinny kids,
Even kids with chicken pox
Love hot dogs, Armour hot dogs
The dogs kids love to bite!

The Vegemite Song

We are happy little Vegemite
As bright as bright can be.
We all enjoy our Vegemite
for breakfast lunch and tea.
Our mommies said we are growing
stronger every single week
Because we love our Vegemite,
We all adore our Vegemite.
It put a rose in every cheek.

Each day we looked forward to exploring new places, meeting new people, and learning about new things; but there were also the ongoing obligations of work and school back home. Often when we left our hotel for meetings with representatives of blindness organizations from throughout the world, David and Dianna would be with us. Dianna looked at the people and the shops. David looked at the cars—especially at a fifty year old Buick, which was frequently parked at the curb. He speculated about the best machine for him, and he remembered that he could only have an automobile of his choice if he kept up his schoolwork. Part of each day was devoted to the study of chemistry, anatomy, English, and history.

We returned to the United States just before Thanksgiving, and we thought about the coming of Christmas. However, David and Dianna discovered that their efforts to maintain their schoolwork while we were away had not kept pace completely with their classes at home, and there was much extra labor in bringing their lessons current.

From time to time David would tell me that he was going to ace his subjects, and I would respond that I hoped he did. I wanted him to do well, but I did not want him to put so much emphasis on the need to do so well that he would feel inadequate or unloved if he did not. I had seen poor grades from him in the past, and I wanted him to know that his mother and I would care for him no less if he did not achieve top marks. We would, of course, be proud of him if his scholarly work was of the first rank, but our love for him is based on something else. Nevertheless, the deal with David demanded top performance before he could receive the reward.

In January the academic quarter for David's high school came to a close, and the report cards were distributed. David is taking six subjects in addition to Junior Seminar. The grades for these subjects, in the quarter completed in January, are all A's.

When he brought me the report card, David said, "You didn't think I could do it, did you?" We are proud of him, and we hope he does it again. If he does, it will be an expensive spring. However, I will get the chance to ride around in a new car. I never expected to buy a new one, but David may be changing my plans. I like cars as much as he does, but I have thought about the matter for a much longer time, and perhaps our perspective is a little different.

He is sighted, and he drives. I am blind, and I do not drive. Nevertheless, I expect to be buying a shiny new car. In the process, I hope that my son will learn just how capable he is. I spend my life working to help blind people know that blindness itself will not prevent success. Hard work and the dream of a better life are essential to building the future that we want.

This is no less true for my sighted son than it is for me, and I want him to believe in his own future as much as I believe in it. And I certainly will be proud to ride with him (at least for a time) on the road to his future successes.

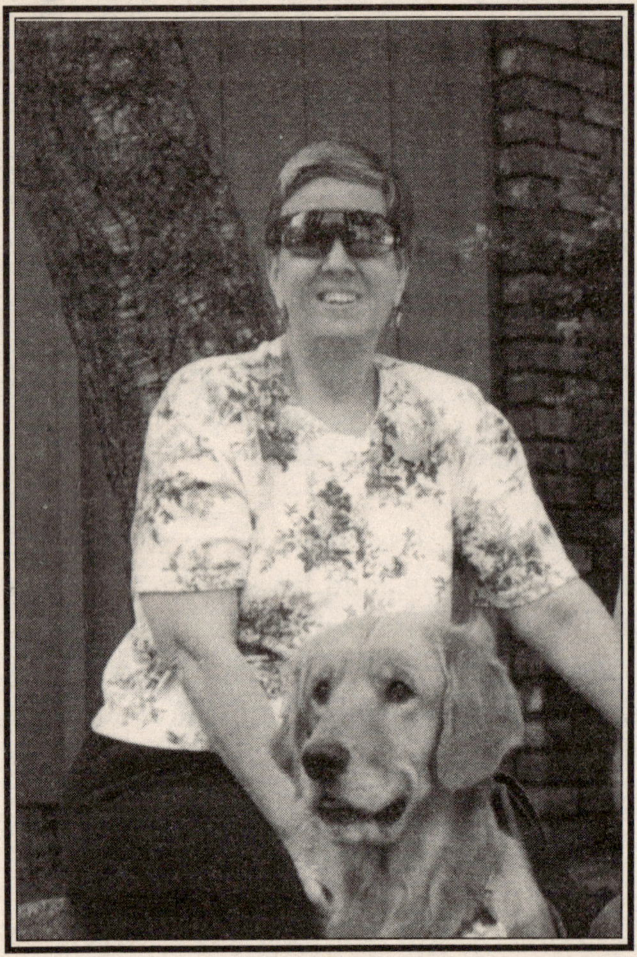

Toni Eames and Ivy

Swimming Was Her Passion!

by Toni Eames

Toni Eames and her husband Ed are longtime members of the National Federation of the Blind. They are professional writers and their work requires them to travel extensively. Both have used guide dogs for many years. In many settings and situations they have written, lectured, and taught about a wide variety of matters relating to blindness and the capacity of blind people to live normal lives.

Imagine their surprise when they learned that one of their most apt pupils had been Toni's guide dog Ivy. It seems that Ivy had been carefully absorbing their lessons over the years, and when she lost her own eyesight, she knew exactly what to do. Here is how Toni tells the story:

I didn't want to face the fact that Ivy, my faithful Golden Retriever guide dog for eleven years, was growing old. Since I could not see the whitening of my Golden girl's muzzle, I was not confronted by the visual image of her aging. She had slowed down, but so had I and we were like perfectly matched book ends.

Over the years, Ivy had developed into a meticulous guide, intuitively recognizing my pervasive fear of losing my balance and falling. Feeling her subtle signals through the harness handle, I confidently negotiated environments as diverse as the subway system in New York City, the buses in Tel Aviv, and major airports throughout the world. Her cautious approach to stairs, curbs, and uneven footing was the hallmark of the effectiveness of our working partnership.

When her caution bordered on hesitancy, I became uneasy and knew there was something drastically wrong. Ivy, the consummate professional, began occasionally failing to stop at curbs and appeared confused when entering a darkened theater from a well-lit lobby.

Fearing for my safety, I consulted with a veterinary ophthalmologist and received the devastating news that Ivy had completely lost vision in one eye. She had continued expertly to perform her duties with such brilliance, I was not even aware she was functioning with limited vision.

Like most Golden Retrievers, Ivy was a glutton. Aside from her insatiable food drive, her other major passion was swimming. It could be a pool, pond, river, or ocean; if it was water Ivy was instinctively drawn to it.

Her love of water first became apparent when I visited my friend Ann Strathurn in Maryland, where strict rules were established about water rights. The pool was for the exclusive use of humans, while the pond was for the canine corps. Shortly after Ivy became my guide, we took a trip to visit Ann. While I cavorted in the pool with Ann's children, Ivy joined Ann's Golden Retrievers in a fenced paddock adjacent to the pool.

Suddenly, I heard a loud splash as Ivy, not recognizing the rules of the house, jumped the five foot fence to get her share of water aerobics. Having been placed back in the paddock, Ivy's water passion was not to be denied! If the pool was off limits, the pond was not!

Jumping the fence in the other direction, Ivy indulged her swimming passion in the designated dog area. For the rest of that visit and subsequent ones, when Ivy was off leash, I allowed her to cavort in the pond.

While Ivy was still working as my guide, but going through vision loss, we revisited the Strathurns. I was surprised to discover the rules at Ann's had been relaxed, and dogs were now invited to join humans in the pool.

During this latest visit, I was concerned that Ivy, with her limited vision, might injure herself trying to get to the water. Not to worry! Since Ivy was familiar with the house and property, she used her residual vision to run around the yard and quickly found the pool. To my dismay, however, when a floating boat bumper was thrown, Ivy dove after it but often swam right by. Eventually scenting the bumper, she retrieved it and brought it to us on the patio.

As dusk fell, Ann noted in distress that Ivy was unable to locate the patio steps and tried to reach us by crashing through the bushes. Ann's observations confirmed my worst fears about Ivy's continuing vision loss and became the basis of her retirement.

By the time Escort, my new Golden Retriever guide dog entered our family, Ivy had become totally blind. Like her human counterparts, she adapted quickly to her blindness, but my emotions were rocked.

The first time she tried to race down the stairs at meal time, she stumbled and slid down several steps. From that time on, she adjusted her pace and never had another close call.

Ivy learned to heel on my right as Escort assumed the guiding role at my left side. Whenever possible, Ivy accompanied me to meetings, restaurants, theater productions, and friends' homes. When my husband Ed and I were away from home overnight, a corps of dog sitters had to be found for Ivy who could not accompany us.

When Helen Shea was the designated dog sitter, Ivy was in ecstasy. Like Ann, Aunt Helen had a pool and dogs were allowed to use it! Although Ivy would have preferred to use the pool throughout the year, she was not allowed to indulge her love of swimming until the weather warmed up.

Finally, that magic day arrived when air and water temperature were right. Like an overprotective parent, something I counsel parents of blind children to avoid, I set about re-introducing Ivy to the pool. Husband Ed, Helen's daughter Beth, and I got into the water and called Ivy to us.

She cautiously negotiated the steps into the pool and swam several feet away. We called her back to the steps, then let her swim further away. After two or three lessons, Ivy demonstrated her confidence by swimming the length of the pool.

Later that afternoon, as we humans dried off on the patio, Ivy emerged from the pool and embarked on an incredible investigation. In awe, Beth described Ivy's movements.

Using her nose as a blind person would use a long white cane, Ivy carefully negotiated the perimeter of the pool, apparently measuring and memorizing the length and width of its boundaries. Having completed her task, she returned to the stairs and effortlessly glided back into her watery haven.

Her message was loud and clear: "You have never allowed your blindness to interfere with your ability to follow your dreams, and adopting your attitude of independence, I too can pursue my passions!"

After-school Homework

by Mark A. Riccobono

Mark Riccobono has been a leader in our organization of blind college students and is now President of the National Federation of the Blind of Wisconsin. If Mark were not blind, the story he tells would not be worth the telling, for there is nothing at all unusual about his experiences as a recent college graduate—which, of course, is exactly the point. Here is what he has to say:

There is much to be said for the college experience. I know. I had as much of it as anybody. In five years of undergraduate work I engaged in many clubs and activities on campus and others off campus, including a semester working in Florida for Walt Disney World and a couple of weeks in England studying international business.

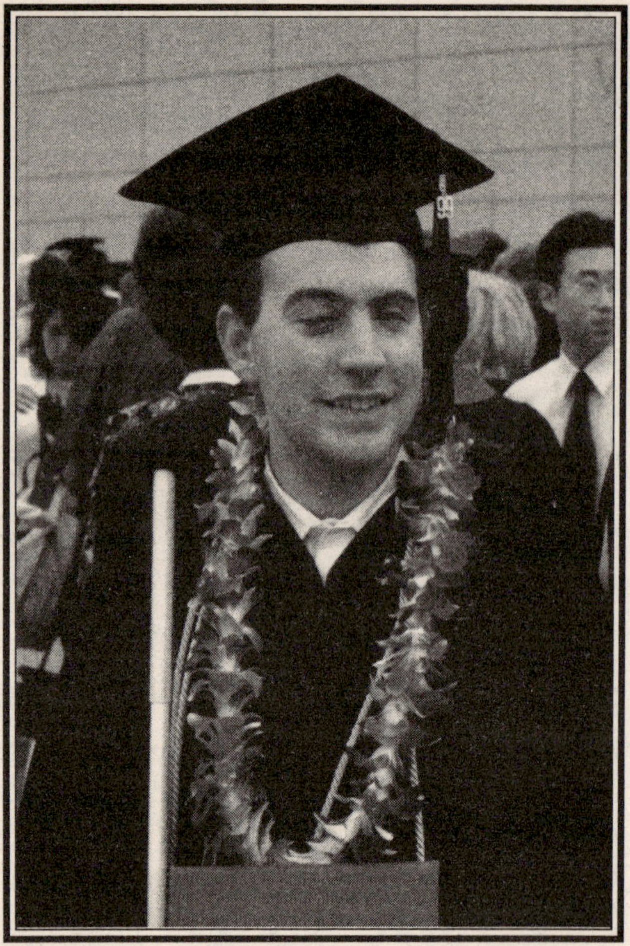

Mark Riccobono

Many people look back at their college years and say that they were the best years of their lives. I have found, in just a few months, that the world after college is more rewarding than one imagines when preparing to leave college.

While college was great, I suspect that the adventures yet to come my way will be increasingly exciting. I believe this because starting my first full-time job has brought many interesting challenges and rewards. However, even more exciting has been beginning to put a home together.

The first step was to find the place. I had grown accustomed to squeezing myself and my few earthly possessions into a small efficiency apartment. Now that I was going to be making real money, that is an income which might actually allow me to accumulate wealth rather than debt, I decided that more space was a high priority.

However, I also know that the long view is important, and I did not want to have to spend so much of my income on rent that I could not save money after all the expenses were paid. Someday I hope to own a house, and it seems to me that some sacrifice and planning today is well worth it. So, I got somebody to help me sort through the piles of apartment listings to find places which met my three basic criteria: cost, space, and location.

Then I began calling around to schedule visits to the prospective new dwellings. When it is convenient I like to take a friend or trusted colleague along to watch for things that I might not notice or remember to ask about and to tell me something about the area, if I am unfamiliar with it. Beyond that, I discuss the details with the landlord, make any appointments or other arrangements, and sign the lease.

I establish from first contact that I am the one looking for the apartment, plan on living by myself, and will make all the payments from money I earn. However, the landlord often does not view the situation that way. The person accompanying me is often thought to be my caretaker, or somebody along those lines, rather than simply a friend.

Often a question is posed like, "What type of amenities is he looking for?" or "Does he have any pets?" I have grown to anticipate this and try to be assertive and respond with kindness, recognizing that many times the landlord is well intentioned.

After a short search (I only had two weeks before I began my new job as a national executive trainee with Sears, Roebuck and Company) I found a comfortable and spacious one-bedroom apartment. Next came the task of filling all that empty space.

As a recent college graduate I had little in the way of furniture and other items which are nice to have in a comfortable home well-suited for living and entertaining guests. I purchased a number of attractive pieces of RTA (ready-to-assemble) furniture. Some people find putting these things together frustrating, but I generally enjoy it, and the fact that I am blind does not affect my ability to complete the job.

Experience is the best teacher. Thus, if you have put RTA furniture together before, you can probably figure it out without reading the instructions, especially if the piece is fairly simple or if you get items by the same manufacturer. I have done it that way before, but I have also had somebody take a few minutes to read the instructions and, if necessary, identify the various pieces by the printed letter on them.

Of course, there is much more to putting a home together: putting up shelves, pictures, and clocks, doing repairs, organizing, arranging, and re-arranging. It can all get very hectic, but it is exciting to be putting together my own little home. I have gotten many compliments from visitors to my home and increasingly enjoy my new home, especially because I have put lots of hard work into it.

There were many times in my life when I wondered what kind of future I could really build for myself. I have often thought that my blindness would prevent me from having the things I wanted to have and doing the things I desired to do—that is, until I won a college scholarship from the National Federation of the Blind of Wisconsin. The money was helpful, but the understanding about blindness and the many people and resources I was exposed to were even more important and continue to be valuable to me.

I learned that it was not my blindness that was going to stop me from reaching my dreams but the misconceptions and negative attitude about blindness which I had learned from society. I quickly found that blindness was neither a blessing nor a tragedy and that my success was dependent on the skills I had and the opportunities I was able to take advantage of. And, more than ever, that is my view today.

There are many people who become blind and assume that they must surrender all of their dreams along with their sight. The National Federation of the Blind has been demonstrating for 60 years that this is not the case. Thanks to my friends in the Federation I did not give up the adventures of "homework" when I graduated from college.

Do You Want to Run?

by Melody Lindsey

Melody Lindsey first became active in the National Federation of the Blind through our scholarship program for blind college students. Today she lives in Michigan where she directs a training center for blind adults. She was part of the delegation attending meetings of the World Blind Union in Melbourne, Australia. While there she journeyed to the "Outback" to visit a sheep farm. Here is what she has to say about her experience there:

As the train pulled out of the Melbourne, Victoria station, it picked up speed quickly. Before long, scenes from the countryside rushed past us almost in a blur. This train was a high-speed train that made stops between Melbourne and Sidney.

The conductor entered the car and began collecting tickets from the passengers. "And where are we going today, Miss?" he asked.

"My destination is The Rock. Can you let me know when we arrive there?" I asked.

"No worries, Mate," he replied jovially. "We should be arriving around 12:30 this afternoon—four hours from now."

A couple minutes later a woman came through the car dispensing tea and other breakfast items. I had never drunk so much tea as I had since arriving in Australia one week earlier. This morning I purchased a cup of tea and settled in for the long trip.

Two days earlier, after the session of the World Blind Union had ended for the day, I began talking to people about the various activities one could do around Australia. I had come to this conference in Melbourne, as a delegate from the United States Rehabilitation Services Administration to

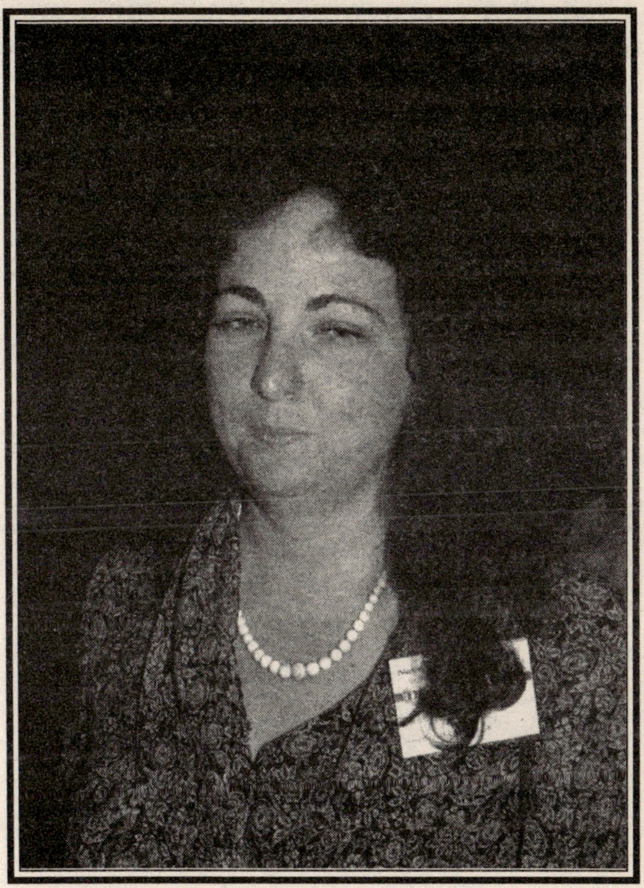

Melody Lindsey

the World Blind Union forum for women. I had a few days in which I could be a tourist and wanted to meet and spend time with everyday Australians.

At dinner that night, a couple attending the meetings of the World Blind Union told me about their itinerary for the next three weeks in Australia. One of the activities that caught my interest was a visit they planned to make to a sheep farm in New South Wales.

The name of the place was Hanericka Farm Stays, and I called the next day to make a reservation. The man who answered the phone took my information and told me to get off the train at the stop called "The Rock."

"Okay," I said. "What is your address so I can tell the cab driver where I need to go?"

The man laughed and informed me that there were no cabs and that they would have someone pick me up from the train.

Next I asked, "Should I call you from the train station?" For some reason I pictured it to be a bustling train station, similar to Melbourne, with numerous telephones and vending machines where a weary traveler could buy coffee or tea.

The man informed me that there were no phones and that all the station would be was a small platform. This was somewhat unsettling to me because, then, what I imagined was a vast desert with one lone train track running through it and a small platform sitting in the midst of rolling sand dunes and tumbleweed. Of course, I imagined poisonous snakes awaiting my arrival under the platform.

In actuality, when I arrived at "The Rock," a young woman named Julie was waiting for me on the platform and introduced herself as the hostess for Hanericka Farm Stays. We got into the car and headed down a two-lane road toward the farm. The train platform was situated in the middle of a small farming community with houses and buildings scattered along the tracks. Oh, and by the way, there were no snakes waiting to greet me either.

When we got to the farmhouse where I would stay, Julie prepared lunch and gave a short tour of the place. I ate lunch with Julie; Yoshi, a farm worker; and Neville, whose children ran various aspects of the farm. It was the end of November, which is the close of spring in Australia. It was very warm and dusty and reminded me of scenes described in Sandy Dengler's Australian Destiny books that I had read a couple of years earlier.

Although the weather was nice, the perpetual presence of swarms of flies was somewhat disconcerting. I was given some spray to deal with these nuisances, which I carried with me almost everywhere I went.

I told Neville the next day at lunch that I had a suggestion for improving the farm. "Oh," he said, "What is it?"

"Get rid of the flies," I said, to which he said that the best way to do that would be to take a dead sheep and put it outside the door so that the flies would be attracted to it and not me. Needless to say, everyone around us thought we engaged in such charming dinner conversation. We did enjoy discussing the American and Australian political systems and other cultural differences and similarities.

After eating breakfast the next morning, Yoshi, who did various chores around the farm, told me that his assignment for the day was to be my tour guide. We went down to the barn and went for a morning ride on two horses. I referred to Yoshi as the Japanese cowboy from Australia because, that's exactly what he was. I asked him why someone from Japan would want to be a cowboy, and then how would that person end up in Australia to follow his dreams. "I always associated cowboys with the Wild West in the United States," I said.

Yoshi was very patient in answering me. "I always loved the open space you find in the outdoors. I liked riding horses and knew that I wanted a job that would combine the two. Japan is a very crowded country with little countryside, so I did some research into cowboy jobs in the United States. There was nothing. But then I learned about a place in Australia that was looking for a farmhand. I applied and came to Australia and have never looked back.

In fact, I am applying for my Australian citizenship because this is where I want to live the rest of my life. I figure I only have one soul, and I should make the best use of it that I can." We then talked about our families and religious beliefs.

After riding in silence for a few minutes, Yoshi asked, "Do you want to run?"

"Can we really?" I asked eagerly.

"Sure," he said, and both of our horses broke into a run. It was so exhilarating to feel the breeze through my hair and to know that someone was not questioning my ability to enjoy a run while on horseback.

It struck me while we were running, "Isn't this what we should be asking blind people who come to us for rehabilitation training? How many times do we prevent people from learning how to run because of our low expectations or our irrational fear of liability ? Blind people should be challenged to learn to run so that they will know that feeling of exhilaration and confidence."

The next day before returning to Melbourne, Yoshi and I went for one last horseback ride. It was more windy on this day, which was both good and bad—good because it kept the flies away and bad because Yoshi and I could not hear each other well.

Yoshi asked, "Do you want to run?" And we took off running across the field.

Suddenly, I heard Yoshi yelling something, but I could not hear him because he was getting farther away. Then, I figured out that my horse must be running the wrong way. It was up to me to get my horse stopped and turned in the right direction—in other words back under control.

Again, I thought, "Isn't this what we should be doing with the blind students who come to us for training? Shouldn't we be teaching them to handle problems that arise independently and competently? And if we always avoid problem situations, how will people learn that they can handle them successfully? Wow," I thought, "Yoshi would make a great teacher!"

That afternoon I left Hanericka Farm Stays feeling that I had made some friends and had learned a great deal about the Australian way of life.

On the train trip back to Melbourne, I reflected on my holiday at the sheep farm.

What had made it so refreshing and invigorating? In recounting the events from the past two days, I decided that what made it such a wonderful vacation was that it was always assumed that I *could* do something.

Of course, there were some people, including the children, who had questions about my blindness, but it seemed to me that they also assumed that I had other interests in addition to blindness. Julie said to me once, "It's good for the kids to spend time around you since they have never seen a blind person. I think that they'll learn that you are not as different as they might think."

I do not know if I will ever get a chance to go back to the sheep farm. I hope so because, since I was there at the end of November and the sheep shearing does not begin until March or April, I have not learned the process involved in shearing a sheep. If I do receive the opportunity, this would be the perfect place to do it because the expectation is there that a blind person not only can do it, but can do it well.

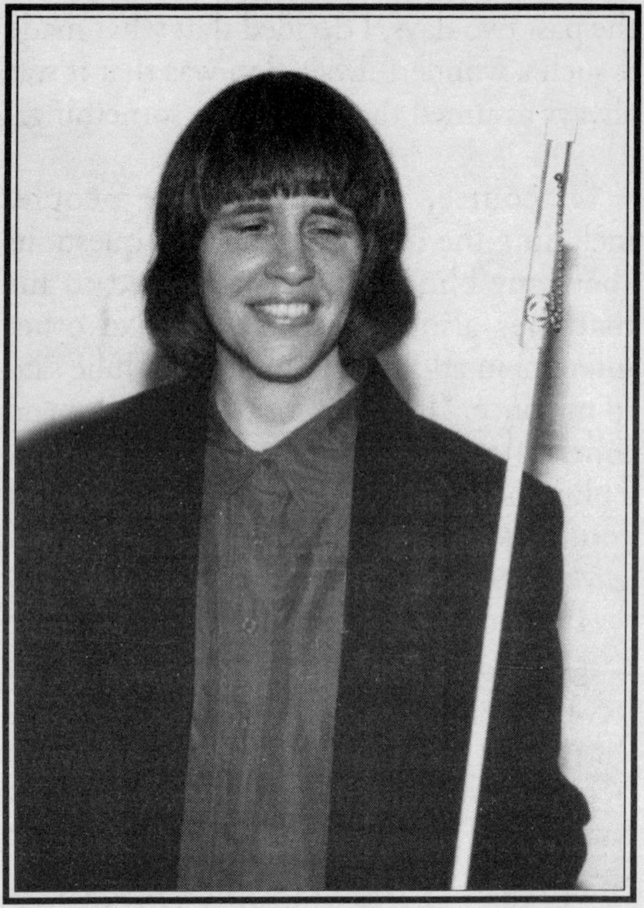

Peggy Elliott

An Unremarkable New Year's Eve

by Peggy Elliott

Peggy Elliott is Second Vice President of the National Federation of the Blind. She is an attorney and serves on the city council in her hometown of Grinnell, Iowa. The story she tells here is quite unremarkable, which, since both she and her husband Doug are blind, is precisely what makes it worth noting. Here is what she has to say:

Everyone has a story about their celebration of the turn-over to the new Millennium. Here's ours:

I serve on the city council, so I knew that staff members of the city government were going to be in the city offices located in our downtown during the turnover in case of problems. In addition, some community-minded women had issued an invitation for everyone in our town to bring hand bells and "ring in the New Year" downtown near a clock that is a replica of one which was located there one hundred years ago.

The mayor was then going to deliver a little address, and we'd all go back home. Not Times Square, but our hometown version of a celebration together.

My husband Doug and I planned a little extra celebration. We took our hand bells and, in addition, a bottle of champagne and some plastic glasses. We figured we'd sneak over to the nearby park after people were gone and have our own little celebration. We turned out to be wrong about that.

The New Year came in. We rang our bells. The mayor gave a graceful little talk. People started to scatter. As we moved onto the sidewalk to start our pretended walk home, we ran into the mayor and one of his friends. We opened the bag slightly, showed what we had, and made a suggestion.

The city manager and city clerk were still on duty. They were being good soldiers, but the fact was that there were no problems to solve. Doug and I suggested that the mayor and his friend accompany us over to the city offices where we would liberate the two city officials and take care of the champagne. Motion carried unanimously.

The problem was that the city offices were locked. I pounded on the steel door with my cane to create a racket while the mayor went round the building into the bushes to try to attract attention by knocking on a window. The manager heard me, and we had to fish the mayor back out of the bushes.

Finally all assembled in the downstairs meeting room, we broke out the bubbly. Doug toasted first, I went second, and the mayor third with a sweet little toast he had learned in our sister city in Russia. We congratulated each other on the uneventful

New Year and went our separate ways, Doug and I walking home through the crisp, cool first hour of the New Year.

Just a sweet little story about what some people in a small Midwestern town decided to do for New Year's Eve. Except for one thing. Doug and I are blind. In our view, this means only that we do some things differently like using our canes instead of our eyes to walk home. But we didn't always feel this way.

Before we met the National Federation of the Blind, we were uncomfortable with our blindness and hesitant to put ourselves forward. Now we know that we are part of our community to the extent of kidnapping the mayor and breaking into the city offices to force champagne on faithful employees.

We not only belong, but we bring champagne and create spontaneous parties. And we believe that the National Federation of the Blind gives us the outlook to do these as well as other, more socially useful things.

I'll Just Give You a Hand

by Barbara Pierce

Barbara Pierce is President of the National Federation of the Blind of Ohio. She is an experienced world traveler and recently was part of the Federation's delegation which attended the meeting of the World Blind Union in Melbourne, Australia.

Here are her thoughtful reflections on the kinds of assistance offered to the blind person out and about in the world. She recognizes the universal good will of those trying to help and the vast differences in skills and training they encounter in the blind people they meet. Here is what she has to say:

I was twelve when I made my first independent airline flight. My parents put me on the plane, and my uncle snagged me at the other end, and I worried during the entire trip of less than an hour about all the things that might go wrong. Like everyone else, in the intervening years I have suffered my share of lost luggage, canceled flights, delays, and last-minute changes in plans. Fortunately for me, I have pretty well stopped worrying about what might go wrong when I travel and how I might cope with the emergency.

As a member of the National Federation of the Blind for more than twenty-five years I have done a lot of flying, and I have met a lot of strangers determined to help me whether I needed assistance or not. Often, of course, I can use a bit of help. When destinations are marked by signs that I can't read, I depend on others to tell me if I am going in the right direction, and I am always grateful for such information.

Several times, however, flight-crew members have demanded that I unfasten my seat belt and refasten it to demonstrate to

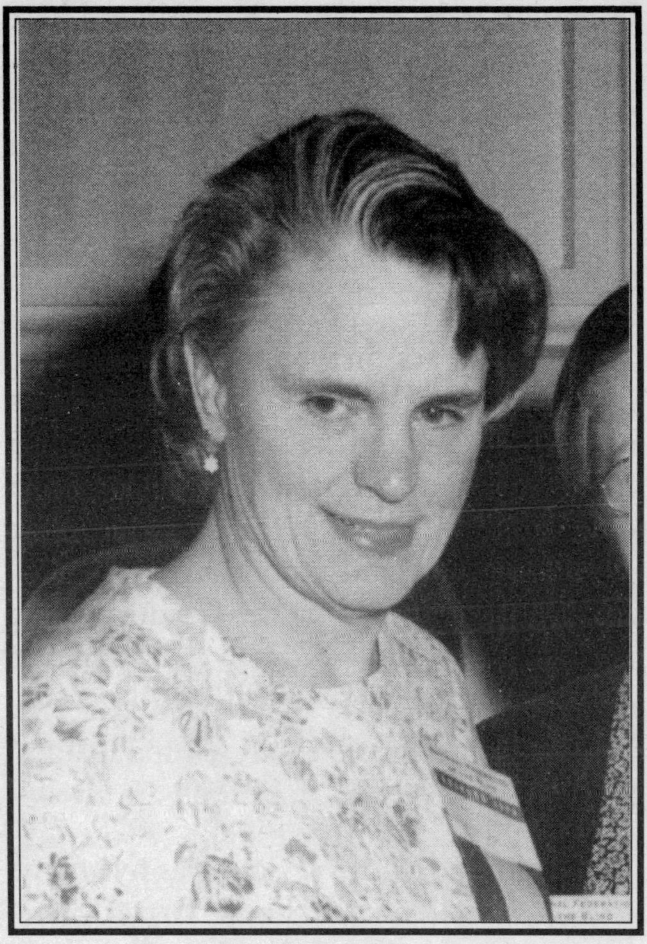

Barbara Pierce

their satisfaction that I can complete the operation independently. Sometimes I have had to insist that an over-zealous crew member tell me where he or she has stashed my luggage after it had been wrenched out of my hands while I was looking for space to stow it myself in the over-head compartment.

Any blind person who travels a lot has to develop ways of dealing with such adventures without becoming annoyed or upset. So when NFB President Marc Maurer called me in early 2000 to tell me that he wanted me to attend a forum in Melbourne, Australia, sponsored by the Committee on the Status of Blind Women of the World Blind Union, I agreed with enthusiasm, wasting no attention on the length or possible complexities of the trip.

I live in the Midwest, so it was five hours to Los Angeles, a five-hour layover there, and a bit over sixteen hours in the air to Melbourne. Several other people attending the same meeting turned out to be on the long leg of my flight, but none was in my section of the plane.

It would be hard to praise the Qantas personnel too highly. They offered to preboard me, but they were also happy to leave me in peace to board when my row was called. When I found my seat, the crew member assigned to the area described the tail section and the location of the rest rooms. She told me exactly where the nearest exits were and offered to answer any other questions.

I took the opportunity to ask about the life vests since I have never been clear about the arrangement of straps, whistle, light, and inflation tube. With no fuss she showed me how the vest works; then she left. I could hardly believe my good luck: a crew member had listened to my questions, answered appropriately, provided useful information, and departed in peace.

The entire flight was filled with more or less the same peace. My seatmates were a pleasant couple vacationing in Australia. Sometimes they talked, and sometimes they read or napped. Some passengers in nearby rows were a bit more intrusive when I went to the rest room, clearly worrying about my ability to get there and back to my seat safely—though I have never been clear about where such people think I am likely to go.

Understandably, when we landed, Qantas wanted to gather all the blind people from the flight together and pass us along to the folks at customs. Since I was not trying to bring illegal substances or products into the country, the customs screening proved to be a simple process.

I did declare a box containing lots of slates and styluses for writing Braille and needles and needle threaders to give as gifts to women in developing countries, but customs officials listened to my explanation, smiled, and passed me along into the warm sunshine of an Australian spring.

The hotel staff were equally willing to offer information or assistance but also happy to leave me to work things out if I wished. American hotels have one great advantage over Australian ones: elevators and rooms here must be labeled in raised print and Braille.

In Australia one had no choice but to count buttons in the elevators and doors on the various floors to get where one wanted to go. But it was all quite manageable, and people consistently provided information if asked for it and went about their business without bothering us if they were not asked.

For the week of my stay I roomed with Melody, another blind woman from the United States, so we very often went places together. We quickly found that Australians on the street were just as sensible as the ones in the hotel. Busy intersections were equipped with quiet clickers to announce when the Walk signs were lighted and when they were not. These were remarkably helpful since the traffic travels on the left, and we sometimes forgot to listen for it in the proper direction.

The audible signals were so quiet that they did not mask traffic sounds, but they did convey what the signs were saying. We found the city very easy to travel in. Trams provided mass transportation. They ran on rails in the center of the street and were remarkably quiet and frequent.

The forum meetings were held in a beautiful old building less than two blocks from our hotel. This was the Melbourne Town Hall. There were lots of steps to climb, both outside and indoors.

Almost all of the delegates and observers to the women's meeting and the larger General Assembly meeting that followed had brought guide/translators with them.

Coming from countries in which not much specialized training is available for blind people, these delegates undoubtedly needed the individual assistance they were using.

All of this help did cause one rather large problem for Melody and me and the handful of other blind people who were not accompanied by their own personal guides. The host organizations had recruited many, many volunteers to help the visitors. You can perhaps begin to understand the nature of the problem.

Any time one of us with a white cane started to go anywhere unaccompanied by a sighted person, we were immediately approached by at least two would-be helpers. That was fine. After all, they had been asked to assist blind people, so they were only doing their job.

The difficulty was that, unlike the many other Australians I was meeting in Melbourne, these folks were determined to take my arm and drag me in the direction they thought I should go. When I asked for directions, I got no answer beyond, "This way; I'll take you."

Both Melody and I found it impossible to explore the building's large entry area in order to master the floor plan. We were simply not allowed to gather information for ourselves, and none of the volunteers would provide it or let anyone else do so without stepping in to provide guide service.

The funniest and most frustrating example of this behavior happened to Melody. She was approaching a curving flight of stairs to the balcony one lunch hour. She arrived at the bottom of the steps at the same moment as a volunteer, who stopped her to point out the hand rail on her right.

Melody, who is young and agile, thanked the woman pleasantly and began climbing the steps without touching the railing.

At that perceived bit of bravado the woman blocked Melody's way with her own body and announced that she was not going to allow Melody to proceed until she took hold of the hand rail. Being acutely aware of the importance of not making a fuss, Melody smiled, placed her right hand on the railing, moved past the woman, and then returned her cane to her right hand once she was safely past the barrier.

Later that day I was waiting for Melody and another friend outside at the corner of the building. They had stayed behind to buy postcards, and we agreed to meet at the corner before deciding what to do next.

I was standing at the exact corner of the building, beside the ramp my friends would come down, at least thirty feet from the intersection. One of the volunteers ran up to me to inquire breathlessly if I was expecting to catch a tram where I was standing. This question provided a good deal of amusement and some insight as well into the minds of the volunteers.

By and large I had found the Australians perfectly ready to provide assistance or not as convenient or requested. They were independent themselves and prepared to assume that other people were equally able to organize their own lives.

The volunteers on the other hand had been asked to help but not, I think, given much direction about what to look for in the people they were offering to assist. Many of the blind visitors needed a great deal of help. They have had no training and are used to being led around and pushed and pulled into position by sighted guides. The poor volunteers didn't know how to deal with people who neither wanted nor needed such treatment.

The National Federation of the Blind has taught me to fight for my own personal independence. But it has also allowed me to observe what happens when people do not have the chance to achieve that independence.

I am deeply grateful that I live in a country in which the general public is coming more and more to recognize the abilities of blind people. I still get plenty of opportunity to practice patience when I travel in the United States, and my sense of humor often holds me in good stead. But as long as I can convince people that I am a responsible adult, I find that by and large, at home or down under, I can handle the people who just want to give me a hand.

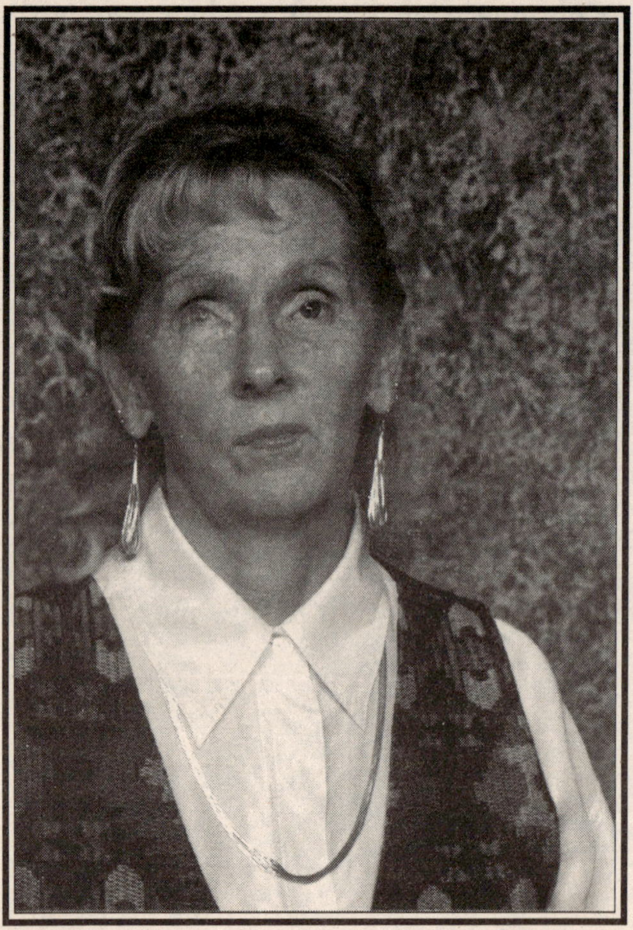

Nancy Burns

Where Do I Go From Here?

by Nancy Burns

Nancy Burns is a long-time leader in the National Federation of the Blind of California. In Where Do I Go From Here? *she tells what it was like to lose her eyesight as an eleven-year-old. Here is what she has to say:*

At the age of eleven I lost my sight, suddenly and traumatically. I had lived with normal vision until that day. I suffered an eye injury which left me totally blind in one eye and with very little sight in the other.

I cannot imagine the grief and shock my family must have experienced, nor could they imagine mine. I truly felt that my life was over. I had no idea where to go or what to do.

This took place in a small, midwestern town. My parents had no knowledge of the National Federation of the Blind or of any support group. We knew no other blind people in the area except for one older, blind couple. I was taken to visit with them but they seemed isolated and different.

After recovering from surgery with no real success, I felt confused and helpless. I don't remember anyone's using the word "blind" in my presence. It was almost that, if it were not discussed, it really did not exist.

Although my life had been drastically changed, deep inside I felt I was still the same little girl. The bad news was that no one else seemed to feel that way.

I was sent back to the public school I had attended prior to my injury. My grandmother attempted to help me catch up with my reading, but I knew it was not going to work. I struggled through school for a few months and finally had to quit. I could not see the blackboard or even the teacher when she stood in front of the windows with the light streaming into the room behind her. I gradually lost the little sight I had retained.

At age thirteen I was sent to the school for the blind in St. Louis, Missouri. The school was residential and was located over 300 miles away from home. Part of me did not want to leave (a big part), but it was the best thing I could have done.

I was amazed to see other blind children running up and down the stairs and through the long corridors of the spacious building. I began to believe that I just might make it as a blind kid after all.

The school for the blind was cxcellent academically. I was taught Braille and was expected to keep up with my classes. I was soon running up and down those same stairs and through the long hallways with my newly found friends. I learned to bowl and roller-skate as a blind child. I participated in home economics classes and learned how to function independently in a kitchen.

I attended social events such as dances, bingo, and card nights. I learned Braille music and took piano lessons as I had done as a sighted kid. I finally came to the realization that I would never be a musician (blind or sighted) and gave the whole thing up.

At the St. Louis school, the word "blind" was certainly used, at least I remember my friends using it. I was still not sure how I would function in the world as a blind person, but I knew that somehow I would. I sort of intellectually learned that being blind was okay, but the emotional or personal aspects of it were still never discussed with me.

My family moved to California just as I was entering the tenth grade. Instead of attending a residential school for blind children, I was mainstreamed into a large public school in Los Angeles. It was a positive transition for me.

In retrospect, I believe I had the best of both worlds, educationally. I gained some real skills and self-confidence at the school for the blind, and I had not been functioning well in the public school.

From high school, I went to UCLA and met some blind students who attended National Federation of the Blind meetings. These were highly motivated blind students, and I liked what they, and the Federation had to say.

"It is respectable to be blind," I was told. Wow! I had finally found a place where blindness could be discussed, and even in a positive manner.

I have spent much of my adult life as an active member of the Federation. I have been supported emotionally by others and, along the way, I have been able to support others in return. I have raised two sighted children and most of this time as a single parent. Being a parent has been a truly rewarding responsibility.

After my boys were out on their own, I returned to school and achieved my master's degree in counseling and psychology. I now operate a home-based consulting business.

I have shared some personal background with you. The purpose of this is to shed some "light" on the word "blind." Also, to point out the importance of positive role models for anyone—blind or sighted.

Although we may seem different to you, we are all just people in the universe. Some of us read print, and some of us read Braille. Some of us drive cars to work, and some of us use public transportation. If we are all grounded in love and understanding, the world will be a better place.

A 3,000-Pound Metallic Puzzle

by Wayne Davis

Wayne Davis is President of the National Federation of the Blind of Florida and a member of the Board of Directors of the National Federation of the Blind. He is also a father and does the things fathers are expected to do—like helping his son with a puzzle—not just an ordinary puzzle but a 3,000-pound metallic one. Here is what he has to say:

My wife Carmen and I are both blind and active members of the National Federation of the Blind. We have a grown son whose name is Dave. At the time of this story David was a senior at the University of South Florida in Tampa.

On the weekend in question Dave had driven home to Miami Beach to spend a little time with us and a great deal of time with his girlfriend Brenda. On his way home on Friday night, he drove through some very heavy South Florida rain, and his windshield wipers had stopped working.

He finally made it home, though, and his very first words when he came into our apartment were, "I am going to fix those blankety-blank windshield wipers first thing in the morning. It won't take more then twenty minutes, and I won't have to spend a lot of money getting it fixed if I do the job myself."

At that time his car was a 1988 Mustang with a 5.0 engine. It had every high-speed add-on that could be put on a car and was only slightly slower than a fighter jet.

I didn't try to talk Dave out of working on his car. To tell the truth, I felt pretty proud

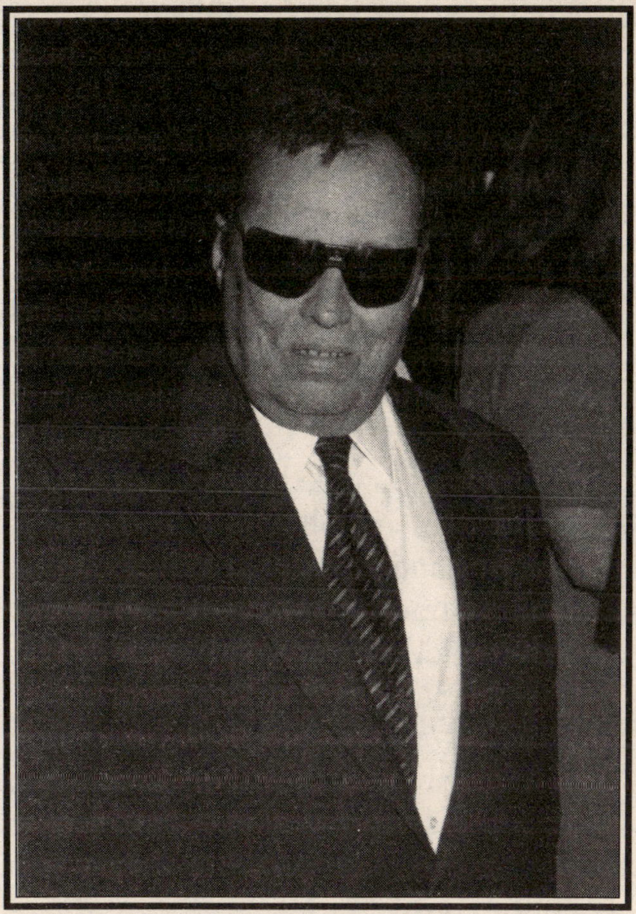

Wayne Davis

of him for being willing to get his hands dirty in order to save a few dollars.

Saturday morning came, and, true to his word, Dave put on an old pair of shorts and went out to fix his windshield wipers. I recall that I was sitting at my computer when I heard him come into the house. "Dad," he said as he leaned against our bedroom door jamb, "Could you help me for a few minutes?"

Fatherly pride swelled my heart. My son, who is a senior in college, needs my help. Here is a chance, I thought, for some of that quality time I am always reading about. "Sure," I said as I slipped on my shoes. "What seems to be the problem?"

"I might have bitten off more than I can chew," he admitted. "I could sure use another pair of hands if you are sure you are not too busy."

"No, Dave," I told him, "What I am doing can wait." Then, like a lamb being led to the slaughter, I followed my son out to the front of our building, where he was working on the car.

"I found out what the problem is," he said. "There are two little holes that let water drain out of the windshield wiper assembly. They are stopped up, and when it rained so hard, water built up and shorted out the wipers." At that point my foot kicked a big metal something lying on the front sidewalk. Before I could even ask, he said sort of under his breath, "That's my left front fender."

"Why did you take off your fender?" I asked.

"It was in the way," he told me, "but that's not my problem, Dad. I can't get my driver's-side door back on by myself."

I tried to remain cool and cling to those earlier thoughts about quality time with my son as I asked him why he had removed his car door.

"Well it wasn't closing right. I had to lift up on it a little to close it sometimes, and I thought I would also fix that problem while I was out here.

"Besides, it was a lot easier to get the fender off once the door was out of the way. It all just sort of got out of hand when I removed those front bolts on the end of the fender. One end of the grill dropped down, and the left headlight sank back toward the radiator. So I went on and just finished taking off the grill. It's lying over by the door and the fender on the sidewalk."

"Dave," I said, as I fought to see the funny side of it all, "Why don't you go into the house and get your mom to give you that large box of trash bags she bought at the grocery store. I'll help you throw the whole thing away."

"Dad," he said, "If I had wanted dumb remarks, I would have just called Brenda. What I want to know is whether we can get it put back together in time for me to make my 2:00 class on Monday afternoon." He went on to tell me that he wanted to beat out a dent or two in the fender he had taken off while he could get to them.

The problem with putting the door back on the car was holding it in just the right position while Dave reattached it. A car door is not particularly light, and with someone else working on it while you are holding it up just so, it quickly gets really heavy.

Moments later, while Dave was inside telling his mom what was going on, a guy pulled up in another Mustang and asked what we were doing. So I told him. He was impressed with all the racing gear and the big souped-up engine.

"What will you take for it?" he inquired. I thought for a second or two and replied: "Is seven dollars too much?" At that moment Dave came hurrying back out to where I was waiting and promptly killed the sale. Somehow, he didn't find that part funny either.

I went to the trunk of his car and got out his jack. After putting my shirt between the jack and the bottom of the car door, I used it to help hold the car door in place until Dave could re-attach the edges.

The fender was another story. It needed more work than we had the tools to do, so we loaded it into the trunk and took it over to an NFB friend's house. Bryan, who is also totally blind, has a shop, and he beat the dents out for Dave and, while he was at it, drilled out some holes for Dave to attach new 5.0 emblems to the fender.

Dave and I both worked all day Saturday and Sunday on the car. We put it back together a piece at a time and did a number of little extra things to it as we went along. We finished up in time for him to make that class on Monday.

He didn't see much of Brenda that weekend, and I wasn't able to get any of my own work done, but I don't think either of us would have swapped that weekend working on that old Mustang for anything.

What does all of this have to do with being blind? Nothing really. That's the whole point. Neither Dave nor I thought my being blind would have any effect on our ability to fix his car. I am his dad, and I have been fixing things around the house since he was born.

He of course knows that Carmen and I are blind, but he also knows that he has always been able to come to either of us with any problem, and the three of us have been able to fix whatever was broken or work out a solution for whatever was wrong.

I am sure he never doubted that together he and I could reassemble his car because he knows that the only difference between us and sighted people is that our eyes don' t work. The rest of us, including our minds and bodies, works just fine.

Even today, five or six years after we put his 3,000-pound model car kit back together, he still calls or stops by to find out what we think about some question he faces in his life. Isn't that what parents are there for?

Members of the National Federation of the Blind are far too busy living our lives to have time to say we can't do something. We may have to develop our own methods of getting it done, but you can rest assured that we will get it done, and it really isn't that big a deal. As in this story, what else could I have done but figure out a way to help Dave fix his car? Sure, I am blind, but after all, I am also his dad.

You can help us spread the word...

...about our Braille Readers Are Leaders contest for blind schoolchildren, a project which encourages blind children to achieve literacy through Braille.

...about our scholarships for deserving blind college students.

...about Job Opportunities for the Blind, a program that matches capable blind people with employers who need their skills.

...about where to turn for accurate information about blindness and the abilities of the blind.

Most importantly, you can help us by sharing what you've learned about blindness in these pages with your family and friends. If you know anyone who needs assistance with the problems of blindness, please write:

Marc Maurer, President
National Federation of the Blind
1800 Johnson Street, Suite 300
Baltimore, Maryland 21230-4998

Other Ways You Can Help the National Federation of the Blind

Write to us for tax-saving information on bequests and planned giving programs.

OR

Include the following language in your will:

"I give, devise, and bequeath unto National Federation of the Blind, 1800 Johnson Street, Suite 300, Baltimore, Maryland 21230, a District of Columbia nonprofit corporation, the sum of $__________ (or "____ percent of my net estate" or "The following stocks and bonds:______") to be used for its worthy purposes on behalf of blind persons."

Your Contributions Are Tax-deductible